Table Of Contents

Chapter 1: Understanding Hair Growth — 4

The Hair Growth Cycle — 4

Factors Affecting Hair Growth — 5

Common Myths about Hair Growth — 6

Chapter 2: Creating the Right Environment for Hair Growth — 8

Proper Scalp Care — 8

Choosing the Right Hair Products — 9

Avoiding Damaging Hair Practices — 10

Chapter 3: Natural Remedies for Fast Hair Growth — 11

Essential Oils for Hair Growth — 11

Homemade Hair Masks and Treatments — 13

Scalp Massages and Stimulating Techniques — 14

Chapter 4: Nutritional Support for Hair Growth — 15

Foods to Eat for Healthy Hair ... 15

Essential Vitamins and Minerals for Hair Growth ... 16

Supplements for Hair Health ... 17

Chapter 5: Lifestyle Habits for Faster Hair Growth ... **19**

Stress Management and its Impact on Hair Growth ... 19

Exercise and its Effect on Hair Health ... 20

Sleep and its Role in Hair Growth ... 21

Chapter 6: Cleaning Methods for Optimal Hair Growth ... **23**

Choosing the Right Shampoo and Conditioner ... 23

How Often to Wash Your Hair for Maximum Growth ... 24

Tips for Proper Hair Washing Techniques ... 25

Chapter 7: Additional Tips and Techniques for Fast Hair Growth ... **27**

Protective Hairstyles for Hair Growth ... 27

Avoiding Heat and Chemical Damage ... 28

How to Deal with Hair Loss and Thinning ... 29

Chapter 8: Maintaining and Managing Fast Hair Growth   **30**

Trimming and Maintaining Hair Length   30

Dealing with Split Ends and Breakage   32

Styling Tips to Showcase Your Fast-Growing Hair   33

Chapter 9: Troubleshooting Hair Growth Issues   **34**

Identifying and Addressing Scalp Conditions   34

Overcoming Hair Growth Plateaus   36

Seeking Professional Help for Hair Growth Concerns   37

Chapter 10: Embracing and Celebrating Your Fast-Growing Hair   **38**

Boosting Confidence and Self-Esteem through Hair Growth   38

Embracing Your Natural Hair Texture   40

Sharing Your Hair Growth Journey with Others   41

Conclusion: Achieving Fast Hair Growth and Maintaining Healthy Hair   **42**

Chapter 1: Understanding Hair Growth

The Hair Growth Cycle

Understanding the hair growth cycle is crucial when it comes to achieving fast hair growth. By familiarizing yourself with the different stages your hair goes through, you can effectively implement the right techniques and remedies to maximize its growth potential. In this subchapter, we will delve into the intricacies of the hair growth cycle and provide you with the knowledge you need to grow your head hair fast.

The hair growth cycle consists of three distinct stages: anagen, catagen, and telogen. The anagen phase is the active growth stage, where your hair follicles produce new cells and push out existing hair strands. This phase typically lasts between two to seven years, and the longer it lasts, the more potential for hair growth you have. Understanding how to prolong the anagen phase is essential for fast hair growth.

Following the anagen phase is the catagen phase, also known as the transitional phase. During this stage, hair growth slows down, and the hair follicles shrink. This phase typically lasts for a few weeks before transitioning into the final stage – the telogen phase.

The telogen phase, also referred to as the resting phase, is when your hair follicles remain inactive for about three to four months. After this period, the old hair strand sheds, and the cycle begins anew. It is important to note that during the telogen phase, new hair begins to grow in the follicles, preparing for the anagen phase once again.

To promote fast hair growth, several techniques and remedies can be implemented. Home remedies such as scalp massages, which stimulate blood flow to the hair follicles, can be highly effective. Additionally, incorporating proper cleaning methods, such as using sulfate-free shampoos and regular scalp exfoliation, can help maintain a healthy scalp environment for optimal hair growth.

Nutrition also plays a vital role in fast hair growth. Consuming a diet rich in essential vitamins and minerals, such as biotin, iron, and vitamin E, can nourish your hair follicles from within, stimulating growth and preventing hair loss. Incorporating foods like eggs, spinach, nuts, and avocados into your diet can provide these necessary nutrients.

In conclusion, understanding the hair growth cycle is essential for anyone seeking fast hair growth. By implementing home remedies, proper cleaning methods, and consuming nutritional foods, you can optimize your hair growth potential and achieve the long, luscious locks you desire. With the knowledge gained in this subchapter, you are equipped with the tools to embark on your journey to fast hair growth.

Factors Affecting Hair Growth

When it comes to growing your head hair fast, there are several factors that can play a significant role in the process. Understanding these factors can help you optimize your hair growth journey and achieve the results you desire. In this subchapter, we will delve into the various factors that affect hair growth and how you can leverage them to stimulate faster hair growth naturally.

1. Genetics: Your genetic makeup plays a crucial role in determining the rate at which your hair grows. While you cannot change your genetics, understanding your hair type and its growth potential can help you set realistic expectations and tailor your hair care routine accordingly.

2. Nutritional Intake: Proper nutrition is essential for healthy hair growth. A diet rich in vitamins, minerals, and proteins can provide the building blocks necessary for strong and fast hair growth. Incorporating foods such as leafy greens, eggs, fish, nuts, and fruits into your diet can contribute to optimal hair health.

3. Scalp Health: A healthy scalp provides the ideal environment for hair growth. Factors such as excessive oiliness, dryness, dandruff, or scalp infections can hinder hair growth. Regularly cleansing your scalp, avoiding harsh chemicals, and maintaining proper hygiene can promote a healthy scalp and stimulate hair growth.

4. Hormonal Balance: Hormonal imbalances, such as thyroid disorders or polycystic ovary syndrome (PCOS), can disrupt the hair growth cycle. If you suspect a hormonal imbalance, it is essential to consult a healthcare professional to address the issue and restore hormonal equilibrium.

5. Stress Levels: High levels of stress can lead to hair loss and hinder hair growth. Practicing stress management techniques, such as meditation, exercise, or engaging in hobbies, can help reduce stress and promote a healthy hair growth environment.

6. Hair Care Routine: The way you care for your hair can significantly impact its growth rate. Avoiding excessive heat styling, using gentle hair products, and minimizing hair breakage by avoiding tight hairstyles can all contribute to faster hair growth.

7. Lifestyle Habits: Certain lifestyle habits, such as smoking, excessive alcohol consumption, and lack of sleep, can negatively impact hair growth. Adopting a healthy lifestyle with adequate sleep, regular exercise, and avoiding harmful habits can support optimal hair growth.

By understanding and addressing these factors, you can create an environment conducive to fast hair growth. In the upcoming chapters, we will explore proven techniques and natural remedies that can further accelerate hair growth, providing you with the ultimate guide to achieving your desired hair length in no time.

Common Myths about Hair Growth

Chapter 3: Common Myths about Hair Growth

Introduction:

In the quest for fast hair growth, it's easy to fall victim to various myths and misconceptions surrounding this topic. While there is no magical overnight solution, understanding the truth behind these common myths will help you make informed decisions on your hair growth journey. In this subchapter, we will debunk some of the most prevalent myths about hair growth and provide you with the facts you need to achieve your desired results.

Myth 1: Cutting your hair frequently makes it grow faster.

One of the most widespread misconceptions is that frequent haircuts stimulate faster hair growth. However, the truth is that hair growth occurs at the follicle, not at the ends. Trimming your hair regularly helps to maintain its health and prevent split ends, but it does not impact the rate of growth.

Myth 2: Brushing your hair 100 times a day promotes faster growth.

While brushing your hair can distribute natural oils and stimulate blood flow to the scalp, excessive brushing can do more harm than good. Over-brushing can lead to hair breakage and damage, hindering your hair growth goals. Instead, opt for gentle brushing techniques and use a wide-toothed comb to detangle your hair.

Myth 3: Shampooing every day is necessary for healthy hair growth.

Contrary to popular belief, washing your hair daily is not essential for fast hair growth. In fact, frequent shampooing can strip away natural oils that are crucial for maintaining healthy hair. Instead, try to wash your hair every two to three days using a gentle, sulfate-free shampoo and conditioner.

Myth 4: Home remedies alone can miraculously accelerate hair growth.

While natural remedies can support hair growth, they are not a magical cure. A holistic approach that combines proper nutrition, scalp care, and a healthy lifestyle is necessary for optimal results. Home remedies, such as applying coconut oil or massaging the scalp with essential oils, can complement your hair growth routine but should not be relied upon solely.

Myth 5: Specific foods can directly increase hair growth speed.

While a balanced diet is essential for overall health, there is no single food that can magically boost hair growth speed. However, certain nutrients like biotin, vitamin E, and omega-3 fatty acids are known to promote healthy hair growth. Incorporating foods rich in these nutrients, such as eggs, nuts, and fatty fish, into your diet can enhance your hair's vitality.

Conclusion:

By debunking these common myths about hair growth, you are now equipped with accurate information to help you achieve your goal of fast hair growth. Remember, patience and consistency are key, along with adopting a comprehensive approach that includes proper hair care, nutrition, and overall wellness. With the right knowledge and dedication, you can unlock the secrets to a luscious and healthy head of hair.

Chapter 2: Creating the Right Environment for Hair Growth

Proper Scalp Care

One of the key factors in achieving fast hair growth lies in taking care of your scalp. Your scalp is the foundation for healthy hair growth, and neglecting it can hinder your progress. This subchapter will guide you through the essential steps of proper scalp care, incorporating both home remedies and effective cleaning methods, along with highlighting the importance of nutritional foods.

Home Remedies for Scalp Care:

1. Scalp Massages: Regularly massaging your scalp stimulates blood circulation, promoting hair growth. Use natural oils like coconut, almond, or olive oil to massage your scalp gently for at least 5-10 minutes before shampooing.

2. DIY Hair Masks: Nourishing your scalp with homemade masks can improve its health and accelerate hair growth. Try mixing ingredients like aloe vera gel, onion juice, egg yolks, and honey to create a potent hair mask. Apply it to your scalp and leave it on for 30 minutes before washing it off.

Effective Cleaning Methods:

1. Choosing the Right Shampoo: Opt for shampoos that are sulfate-free, as sulfates can strip your scalp of its natural oils, leading to dryness and hair damage. Look for shampoos containing natural ingredients like aloe vera, tea tree oil, or rosemary, which can promote a healthy scalp.

2. Regular Cleansing: Cleanse your scalp and hair regularly to remove dirt, excess oil, and product buildup. However, avoid over-washing, as it can strip away essential oils, causing dryness. Find a balance that suits your scalp type, whether it's washing every other day or a couple of times a week.

Nutritional Foods for a Healthy Scalp:

1. Omega-3 Fatty Acids: Incorporate foods rich in omega-3 fatty acids such as fatty fish (salmon, mackerel), chia seeds, flaxseeds, and walnuts into your diet. These healthy fats nourish the scalp and support hair growth.

2. Biotin-Rich Foods: Consume foods like eggs, nuts, spinach, and avocados that are high in biotin, a B-vitamin essential for healthy hair growth and scalp health.

Remember, the health of your scalp is directly linked to the growth of your hair. By following these proper scalp care techniques, you can create an optimal environment for your hair to grow faster and healthier.

Choosing the Right Hair Products

When it comes to achieving fast hair growth, it's not just about using home remedies and nutritional foods. The hair products you choose can play a significant role in promoting healthy hair growth. With a plethora of options available in the market, it can be overwhelming to select the right ones. This subchapter will guide you through the process of choosing the best hair products that will support your goal of growing your head hair fast.

First and foremost, it is important to understand your hair type and its specific needs. Is your hair dry, oily, or prone to frizz? Identifying these characteristics will help you select products that cater to your hair's unique requirements. For instance, if you have dry hair, look for moisturizing shampoos and conditioners that will nourish and hydrate your locks.

Additionally, pay attention to the ingredients list. Avoid products that contain harsh chemicals such as sulfates and parabens, as they can strip your hair of its natural oils and hinder its growth. Instead, opt for products that are free from these harmful substances and enriched with natural ingredients like aloe vera, coconut oil, and argan oil.

Consider investing in a good-quality shampoo and conditioner specifically formulated for promoting hair growth. Look for products that contain ingredients known to stimulate the hair follicles and improve blood circulation to the scalp. Examples of such ingredients include biotin, keratin, and vitamins A, C, and E.

In addition to shampoos and conditioners, incorporate other hair care essentials into your routine. A wide-toothed comb or a brush with soft bristles will help detangle your hair gently, preventing breakage. Furthermore, using a heat protectant spray before styling with hot tools can prevent damage and preserve the health of your hair.

Lastly, don't forget to consider your own preferences and lifestyle. If you prefer a particular scent or texture, choose products that align with your personal tastes. Additionally, if you lead an active lifestyle and frequently engage in physical activities, opt for products that are designed to withstand sweat and humidity.

By carefully selecting the right hair products, you can provide your hair with the necessary nourishment and care it needs to grow faster and healthier. Remember, growing your head hair fast is not just about what you put inside your body, but also what you put on it.

Avoiding Damaging Hair Practices

Growing your hair fast is not just about using the right home remedies and nutritional foods; it also involves avoiding damaging hair practices. In this subchapter, we will explore some common practices that can hinder hair growth and provide you with valuable tips on how to steer clear of them.

1. Overstyling: Excessive use of heat styling tools such as straighteners, curling irons, and blow dryers can damage your hair, making it weak and prone to breakage. Limit the use of these tools and opt for heat-free styling techniques whenever possible.

2. Tight Hairstyles: Wearing your hair in tight ponytails, braids, or buns can cause tension on your scalp, leading to hair breakage and traction alopecia. Allow your hair to breathe by opting for loose hairstyles and avoiding tight hair accessories.

3. Chemical Treatments: Frequent use of chemical treatments like relaxers, perms, and hair dyes can cause significant damage to your hair. Opt for natural alternatives or consult a professional stylist to minimize the harm caused by these treatments.

4. Rough Towel Drying: Vigorously rubbing your hair with a towel after washing can lead to hair breakage and frizz. Instead, gently squeeze out the excess water and allow your hair to air dry or use a microfiber towel to minimize damage.

5. Harsh Shampooing: Using harsh shampoos that contain sulfates and other harsh chemicals can strip away natural oils from your hair, making it dry and brittle. Look for sulfate-free and gentle shampoos that promote hair health.

6. Overwashing: Washing your hair too frequently can strip away essential oils, leading to dryness and damage. Aim for washing your hair every two to three days or as needed to maintain a healthy balance.

7. Neglecting Scalp Health: A healthy scalp is essential for hair growth. Avoid neglecting your scalp by regularly massaging it with natural oils, exfoliating to remove dead skin cells, and maintaining good hygiene.

By avoiding these damaging hair practices, you can create an optimal environment for fast hair growth. Remember, growing your hair requires a holistic approach that encompasses both the right practices and the avoidance of damaging ones. With the right knowledge and commitment, you can achieve the luscious locks you desire.

Chapter 3: Natural Remedies for Fast Hair Growth

Essential Oils for Hair Growth

When it comes to growing your head hair fast, natural remedies are often the best solution. One such remedy that has gained significant popularity in recent years is the use of essential oils. Packed with nutrients and powerful properties, essential oils can help nourish your scalp, strengthen your hair follicles, and promote hair growth. In this subchapter, we will explore the top essential oils for hair growth and how to use them effectively.

1. Rosemary Oil:

Known for its stimulating properties, rosemary oil is excellent for improving blood circulation in the scalp, which in turn promotes hair growth. To use rosemary oil, simply mix a few drops with a carrier oil such as coconut or jojoba oil, and massage it into your scalp. Leave it on for at least 30 minutes before rinsing it off.

2. Lavender Oil:

Lavender oil not only has a calming aroma but also helps to balance the natural oils on your scalp. This oil is particularly beneficial for those with dry or itchy scalps. Mix a few drops of lavender oil with a carrier oil and apply it to your scalp. Leave it on overnight for best results.

3. Peppermint Oil:

Peppermint oil is known for its cooling and soothing effects. It can help relieve scalp irritation and stimulate hair growth. Mix a few drops of peppermint oil with a carrier oil and massage it into your scalp. Leave it on for 15-20 minutes before rinsing it off.

4. Cedarwood Oil:

Cedarwood oil has been used for centuries to treat hair loss and promote hair growth. It helps balance oil production, stimulates the scalp, and strengthens hair follicles. Mix a few drops of cedarwood oil with a carrier oil and apply it to your scalp. Leave it on overnight and wash it off in the morning.

5. Tea Tree Oil:

Tea tree oil is well-known for its antifungal and antibacterial properties, making it effective in treating scalp conditions that may hinder hair growth. Mix a few drops of tea tree oil with a carrier oil and massage it into your scalp. Leave it on for 30 minutes before rinsing it off.

Remember to always dilute essential oils with a carrier oil before applying them to your scalp. Also, conduct a patch test to check for any allergic reactions. Consistency is key when using essential oils for hair growth, so make it a part of your regular hair care routine. With the right combination of essential oils and proper hair care techniques, you can achieve faster hair growth naturally.

Homemade Hair Masks and Treatments

When it comes to achieving fast hair growth, homemade hair masks and treatments can be incredibly effective. Not only are these remedies natural and chemical-free, but they can also be easily prepared at home using common ingredients found in your kitchen pantry. In this subchapter, we will explore some of the best homemade hair masks and treatments that can promote rapid hair growth.

1. Coconut Oil and Honey Mask: Coconut oil is known for its moisturizing properties, while honey helps to nourish the scalp and stimulate hair growth. To create this mask, mix equal parts of coconut oil and honey and apply it to your hair from root to tip. Leave it on for 30 minutes before rinsing it off with a mild shampoo.

2. Egg and Yogurt Hair Mask: Eggs are rich in protein, which is essential for promoting hair growth, while yogurt helps to condition and strengthen the hair. Blend one egg with two tablespoons of plain yogurt and apply the mixture to your hair. Leave it on for 20 minutes before washing it off with lukewarm water.

3. Avocado and Olive Oil Treatment: Avocado is packed with vitamins and minerals that nourish the scalp and promote hair growth, while olive oil adds moisture and shine to your locks. Mash a ripe avocado and mix it with two tablespoons of olive oil. Apply the mixture to your hair, focusing on the roots, and leave it on for 30 minutes before rinsing it off.

4. Aloe Vera Gel Scalp Treatment: Aloe vera is known for its soothing and moisturizing properties, making it an excellent treatment for a dry and itchy scalp. Apply aloe vera gel directly to your scalp and massage it gently for a few minutes. Leave it on for an hour before rinsing it off with a mild shampoo.

5. Onion Juice Rinse: Onion juice is rich in sulfur, which promotes hair growth and reduces hair fall. Extract the juice from an onion and apply it to your scalp. Leave it on for 15 minutes before rinsing it off with a gentle shampoo.

By incorporating these homemade hair masks and treatments into your hair care routine, you can nourish your scalp, strengthen your hair follicles, and stimulate fast hair growth naturally. Remember to be consistent with these remedies and combine them with a healthy diet and proper hair care practices for the best results.

Scalp Massages and Stimulating Techniques

A key aspect of achieving fast hair growth lies in taking care of your scalp. By implementing scalp massages and stimulating techniques into your hair care routine, you can promote increased blood circulation, nourish hair follicles, and accelerate hair growth naturally. In this subchapter, we will explore how scalp massages and stimulating techniques can be effective tools for achieving the luscious locks you desire.

Scalp massages have been used for centuries as a method to stimulate hair growth. The gentle pressure applied during a scalp massage helps to increase blood flow to the hair follicles, providing them with essential nutrients and oxygen. Additionally, the massaging action helps to relax the scalp, reducing stress and tension, which can contribute to hair loss.

To perform a scalp massage, start by using your fingertips to apply gentle pressure to your scalp in circular motions. Begin at the front of your head and move towards the back, covering the entire scalp. You can use a natural oil, such as coconut or jojoba oil, to enhance the massage and provide additional nourishment to your scalp and hair.

In addition to scalp massages, there are various stimulating techniques that can promote fast hair growth. One such technique is known as scalp tapping. Using your fingertips or a soft brush, lightly tap your scalp all over, focusing on areas where hair growth is desired. This tapping motion helps to stimulate blood circulation and awaken dormant hair follicles.

Another effective technique is called inversion therapy. By hanging your head upside down for a few minutes each day, either by using an inversion table or simply bending over, you can increase blood flow to the scalp. This increased blood flow nourishes the hair follicles and encourages hair growth.

It is important to note that while scalp massages and stimulating techniques can be beneficial, they are most effective when combined with a holistic approach to hair care. This includes adopting a nutritious diet, using natural hair care products, and practicing good hygiene.

In summary, incorporating scalp massages and stimulating techniques into your hair care routine can be a powerful tool in achieving fast hair growth. These techniques help to increase blood circulation, nourish hair follicles, and reduce stress, all of which contribute to healthy hair growth. By embracing these natural remedies, cleaning methods, and nutritional foods, you can unlock the secrets to growing long, beautiful hair from the comfort of your own home.

Chapter 4: Nutritional Support for Hair Growth

Foods to Eat for Healthy Hair

When it comes to achieving fast hair growth, you may have already tried various home remedies and cleaning methods. However, did you know that the food you eat plays a crucial role in promoting healthy hair growth? In this subchapter, we will explore the nutritional foods that can help you achieve your desired results.

1. Protein-rich foods: Your hair is primarily composed of protein, so it's essential to include adequate amounts in your diet. Incorporate lean meats such as chicken, turkey, and fish, or opt for plant-based sources such as lentils, beans, and tofu. These foods provide the necessary amino acids that promote hair growth and strength.

2. Omega-3 fatty acids: Found in abundance in fatty fish like salmon, mackerel, and sardines, omega-3 fatty acids are essential for maintaining a healthy scalp and promoting hair growth. If you're vegetarian or vegan, you can try incorporating flaxseeds, chia seeds, or walnuts into your diet as alternative sources of these beneficial fats.

3. Vitamins and antioxidants: Certain vitamins and antioxidants are crucial for healthy hair growth. Vitamin A, found in carrots, sweet potatoes, and spinach, helps produce sebum, which moisturizes the scalp and keeps your hair healthy. Vitamin C, abundant in citrus fruits and berries, aids in collagen production, promoting hair strength. Additionally, vitamin E-rich foods like almonds and avocados protect your hair from damage caused by free radicals.

4. Biotin-rich foods: Biotin, a B-vitamin, is often associated with hair growth. Include foods like eggs, nuts, seeds, and leafy greens in your diet to ensure an adequate intake of biotin.

5. Iron and zinc: Both iron and zinc deficiencies can lead to hair loss and slow hair growth. Consume iron-rich foods such as lean red meat, spinach, and lentils. Zinc can be found in oysters, shellfish, pumpkin seeds, and beef.

Remember, while incorporating these hair-friendly foods into your diet, it's also essential to maintain a balanced eating plan overall. Hydration is equally important, so ensure you're drinking enough water to keep your hair and scalp hydrated.

By incorporating these nutritional foods into your diet, you are providing your body with the necessary building blocks for healthy hair growth. Combine these dietary changes with the techniques and natural remedies discussed in this book, and you'll be well on your way to achieving fast hair growth and maintaining luscious locks.

Essential Vitamins and Minerals for Hair Growth

When it comes to achieving fast hair growth, there are several key vitamins and minerals that play a crucial role in promoting healthy hair. By incorporating these nutrients into your diet, you can nourish your hair from within and support its growth. In this subchapter, we will explore the essential vitamins and minerals that can help you achieve the luscious locks you desire.

1. Vitamin A: This vitamin is essential for maintaining a healthy scalp. It promotes the production of sebum, the natural oil that keeps your scalp moisturized. Foods rich in vitamin A include carrots, sweet potatoes, and spinach.

The Ultimate Guide to Fast Hair Growth: Proven Techniques and Natural Remedies

2. Biotin: Also known as vitamin B7, biotin is often referred to as the "hair growth vitamin." It aids in the production of keratin, a protein that forms the structure of your hair. Sources of biotin include eggs, nuts, and whole grains.

3. Vitamin C: This antioxidant vitamin strengthens the hair shaft and prevents breakage. It also aids in the absorption of iron, which is crucial for hair growth. Citrus fruits, strawberries, and bell peppers are excellent sources of vitamin C.

4. Vitamin E: Known for its antioxidant properties, vitamin E improves blood circulation to the scalp, promoting hair growth. Include foods like almonds, avocados, and sunflower seeds in your diet to boost your vitamin E intake.

5. Iron: Iron deficiency can lead to hair loss, making it vital to include iron-rich foods such as lean meats, spinach, and lentils in your diet. Iron helps carry oxygen to the hair follicles, stimulating hair growth.

6. Zinc: This mineral plays a crucial role in hair tissue growth and repair. It helps maintain the oil glands around the hair follicles, preventing dryness and dandruff. Oysters, beef, and pumpkin seeds are excellent sources of zinc.

By ensuring you have an adequate intake of these essential vitamins and minerals, you can provide your hair with the necessary building blocks for fast growth. However, it is important to remember that while nutritional support is crucial, external hair care practices and overall health also contribute to the hair growth process. Therefore, it is recommended to combine these dietary changes with proper hair care techniques and a healthy lifestyle to maximize the results.

In the following chapters, we will dive deeper into home remedies, cleaning methods, and nutritional foods that can further enhance your hair growth journey. With the right combination of internal and external care, you can achieve the fast hair growth you desire and enjoy a head full of healthy, vibrant locks.

Supplements for Hair Health

In our quest for fast hair growth, we often tend to overlook the importance of nourishing our hair from within. While external treatments and home remedies have their place, it is crucial to understand that our hair's health largely depends on the nutrients we provide our bodies. This subchapter will explore the role of supplements in promoting hair growth and enhancing overall hair health.

1. Biotin: Known as the "hair growth vitamin," biotin is a B-complex vitamin that plays a vital role in the production of keratin, the protein that constitutes our hair. By taking biotin supplements, you can strengthen your hair follicles, prevent hair breakage, and encourage healthy growth.

2. Vitamin E: This powerful antioxidant not only boosts blood circulation to the scalp but also helps in repairing damaged hair follicles. By incorporating vitamin E supplements into your routine, you can promote hair growth and improve hair texture.

3. Omega-3 Fatty Acids: Found in fish oil supplements, omega-3 fatty acids are essential for maintaining a healthy scalp and hair. These fatty acids nourish the hair follicles, reduce inflammation, and prevent dryness and flakiness, leading to faster hair growth.

4. Iron: Iron deficiency is a common cause of hair loss and slow hair growth. Supplementing with iron can help replenish iron stores in the body, enhance oxygen flow to the scalp, and stimulate hair growth.

5. Zinc: This mineral is crucial for maintaining a healthy scalp and preventing hair loss. Zinc supplements can regulate oil production, strengthen hair follicles, and boost hair growth.

6. Vitamin D: Research suggests that vitamin D deficiency may contribute to hair loss. By taking vitamin D supplements, you can ensure that your hair follicles receive the necessary nutrients for optimal growth.

7. Multivitamins: While specific vitamins and minerals are essential for hair health, it is important to maintain overall nutritional balance. A good-quality multivitamin can provide a comprehensive range of vitamins and minerals, ensuring that your body has all the necessary nutrients for healthy hair growth.

Remember, supplements should be used in conjunction with a healthy diet and lifestyle. It is always advisable to consult with a healthcare professional before starting any new supplements, as they can provide personalized guidance based on your unique needs.

By incorporating these supplements into your daily routine, you can provide your hair with the vital nourishment it needs for fast hair growth and improved overall hair health.

Chapter 5: Lifestyle Habits for Faster Hair Growth

Stress Management and its Impact on Hair Growth

In our fast-paced, modern lives, stress has become an inevitable part of our daily routine. This constant pressure not only affects our mental and physical well-being but can also have a significant impact on our hair growth. Understanding the connection between stress and hair growth is crucial for anyone seeking to achieve fast hair growth on their head.

When we experience stress, our bodies release hormones like cortisol and adrenaline. While these hormones are essential for our survival, prolonged exposure to high levels of stress can disrupt the natural hair growth cycle. Stress can lead to hair loss, thinning, and even a delay in the growth of new hair.

One of the ways stress affects hair growth is by pushing hair follicles into a resting phase, known as telogen effluvium. This condition can cause a significant amount of hair to shed at once, leaving individuals with noticeable thinning or bald patches. Additionally, stress can also disrupt the production of keratin, a protein essential for hair growth, leading to weaker and slower-growing hair strands.

Fortunately, there are various stress management techniques that can help mitigate the effects of stress on hair growth. Firstly, it is crucial to identify the sources of stress in your life and find healthy ways to manage them. This might involve incorporating relaxation techniques such as meditation, deep breathing exercises, or yoga into your daily routine.

Regular exercise is another effective stress management tool. Engaging in physical activities like jogging, swimming, or cycling not only helps reduce stress levels but also improves blood circulation, delivering essential nutrients to the hair follicles and promoting hair growth.

Nutrition also plays a vital role in combating the effects of stress on hair growth. A balanced diet rich in vitamins, minerals, and proteins can provide the necessary building blocks for healthy hair. Incorporating foods like eggs, fish, spinach, nuts, and avocados into your meals can help nourish your hair from within.

Furthermore, it is important to create a self-care routine that prioritizes relaxation and rejuvenation. This might include indulging in scalp massages, using natural remedies like essential oils, and adopting gentle hair care practices that minimize damage to your hair follicles.

By managing stress effectively and adopting healthy lifestyle choices, you can significantly improve your hair growth rate. Remember, achieving fast hair growth on your head requires a holistic approach that addresses not only external factors but also internal well-being. Take charge of your stress levels, nourish your body with the right nutrients, and watch your hair flourish like never before.

Exercise and its Effect on Hair Health

Introduction:

In our pursuit of fast hair growth, it is essential to explore all the factors that contribute to healthy hair. While we often focus on external factors such as home remedies, cleaning methods, and nutritional foods, we tend to overlook the impact that exercise has on our hair health. In this subchapter, we will delve into the connection between exercise and hair growth, uncovering the benefits of physical activity for a luscious and vibrant mane.

The Link between Exercise and Hair Growth:

Regular exercise not only promotes overall well-being but also has a profound impact on hair health. Engaging in physical activity stimulates blood circulation, ensuring that essential nutrients and oxygen reach the hair follicles. This enhanced blood flow nourishes the hair roots, subsequently promoting hair growth and preventing hair loss. Additionally, exercise helps regulate hormonal balance, reducing the likelihood of hair thinning and shedding.

Types of Exercise for Optimal Hair Health:

While any form of physical activity is beneficial for hair growth, certain exercises have proven to be particularly effective. Cardiovascular exercises such as running, cycling, and swimming increase heart rate and improve blood circulation throughout the body, including the scalp. Strength training exercises, such as weightlifting and yoga, also play a significant role in hair health by reducing stress levels and balancing hormones.

Precautions to Consider:

While exercise is generally beneficial for hair health, certain precautions should be taken to avoid causing damage. Excessive sweating can lead to a build-up of sebum and dirt on the scalp, potentially clogging hair follicles and hindering hair growth. To combat this, it is crucial to maintain proper hygiene by washing the hair regularly and using suitable hair products. Additionally, protecting the hair from excessive friction and pulling during exercise, especially for individuals with long hair, is essential to prevent breakage.

Conclusion:

In our quest for fast hair growth, it is crucial to recognize the role that exercise plays in promoting hair health. By incorporating regular physical activity into our routines, we can improve blood circulation, nourish hair follicles, and maintain hormonal balance – all of which are vital for achieving long, healthy hair. However, it is essential to exercise caution and maintain proper hygiene to prevent any potential damage. Remember, exercise is not only beneficial for our bodies but also for our hair, offering us a holistic approach to achieving our hair growth goals.

Sleep and its Role in Hair Growth

Getting a good night's sleep is not only crucial for our overall well-being but also plays a significant role in the growth and health of our hair. In this subchapter, we will explore the connection between sleep and hair growth, providing you with valuable insights and tips on how to optimize your sleep to promote fast hair growth.

Quality sleep is essential for the body to repair and rejuvenate itself. During the sleep cycle, our body releases growth hormones that stimulate cell regeneration and repair damaged tissues, including hair follicles. Lack of sleep or poor sleep quality can disrupt this natural process, leading to impaired hair growth and potential hair loss.

One of the key factors affecting sleep quality is the hormone melatonin. Known as the "sleep hormone," melatonin regulates our sleep-wake cycle. Studies have shown that melatonin also plays a role in hair growth by promoting hair follicle development and preventing hair loss. To ensure optimal melatonin production, it is important to establish a consistent sleep routine and create a sleep-friendly environment, including a dark, quiet, and comfortable bedroom.

In addition to melatonin, sleep deprivation can also lead to increased levels of stress hormones such as cortisol. Elevated cortisol levels can negatively impact hair growth by disrupting the hair follicle's natural cycle and triggering hair loss. Therefore, managing stress and prioritizing sleep are essential for maintaining healthy hair growth.

To promote fast hair growth through optimal sleep, here are some practical tips:

1. Create a Relaxing Bedtime Routine: Establish a calming routine before bed, such as reading a book, taking a warm bath, or practicing meditation. This will signal your body that it's time to wind down and prepare for sleep.

2. Maintain a Consistent Sleep Schedule: Try to go to bed and wake up at the same time every day, even on weekends. Consistency helps regulate your body's internal clock and promotes better sleep quality.

3. Invest in a Comfortable Mattress and Pillow: A supportive mattress and pillow can improve your sleep posture, reducing the risk of hair breakage and promoting healthy hair growth.

4. Avoid Stimulants and Electronic Devices: Limit the consumption of caffeine, nicotine, and alcohol before bedtime, as they can disrupt sleep patterns. Additionally, avoid using electronic devices like smartphones and laptops, as the blue light emitted can interfere with melatonin production.

By incorporating these sleep-enhancing practices into your daily routine, you can harness the power of quality sleep to boost your hair growth efforts. Remember, the path to fast hair growth starts with taking care of your body, and sleep is an integral part of that process.

Chapter 6: Cleaning Methods for Optimal Hair Growth

Choosing the Right Shampoo and Conditioner

When it comes to achieving fast hair growth, choosing the right shampoo and conditioner can play a crucial role. These hair care products are not only responsible for cleansing and conditioning your hair, but they also contribute to its overall health and vitality. In this subchapter, we will explore the key factors to consider when selecting the perfect shampoo and conditioner for promoting fast hair growth.

Firstly, it is essential to understand your hair type and its specific needs. Different hair types require different care, and using the wrong products can hinder your hair growth goals. Whether you have oily, dry, or combination hair, opt for shampoos and conditioners that are specifically formulated for your hair type. Look for products that provide moisture, hydration, and nourishment without weighing your hair down or causing excessive dryness.

Another important consideration is to choose shampoos and conditioners that are free from harsh chemicals and sulfates. These ingredients can strip your hair of its natural oils, leading to dryness and damage. Instead, opt for natural and organic products that are gentle on your scalp and hair. Look for ingredients like aloe vera, argan oil, and coconut oil, which promote hair growth and provide essential nutrients.

Furthermore, pay attention to the specific ingredients that target hair growth. Look for shampoos and conditioners that contain biotin, keratin, and vitamins like B and E. These ingredients stimulate hair follicles, strengthen the hair shaft, and promote healthy growth. Additionally, products infused with essential oils such as rosemary, lavender, and peppermint can also enhance blood circulation to the scalp, stimulating hair growth.

Consider the pH level of the shampoo and conditioner you choose. A slightly acidic pH, around 5.5, is ideal for maintaining the health and balance of your scalp. This pH level helps to retain moisture and prevent scalp issues, which can hinder hair growth.

Finally, be consistent with your hair care routine. Use the chosen shampoo and conditioner regularly, preferably every other day or as instructed on the product label. Consistency is key to achieving fast hair growth and reaping the benefits of the chosen products.

In conclusion, selecting the right shampoo and conditioner is a vital step towards achieving fast hair growth. By considering your hair type, opting for natural ingredients, and looking for specific growth-promoting ingredients, you can optimize your hair care routine. Remember to be consistent and patient, as healthy hair growth takes time. With the right products, dedication, and a holistic approach, you can unlock the secrets to fast hair growth and enjoy a head full of beautiful, healthy hair.

How Often to Wash Your Hair for Maximum Growth

One of the keys to achieving fast hair growth lies in maintaining a proper hair care routine. While there are numerous factors that contribute to hair growth, such as genetics, diet, and overall health, it is crucial to pay attention to how often you wash your hair. In this subchapter, we will delve into the topic of how frequently you should wash your hair for maximum growth, providing you with proven techniques and natural remedies to accelerate the growth process.

The frequency of washing your hair primarily depends on your hair type and scalp condition. For those aiming to grow their head hair fast, it is generally recommended to wash your hair every two to three days. This interval allows the natural oils produced by your scalp, known as sebum, to nourish and moisturize your hair. Overwashing can strip away these essential oils, leading to dryness and breakage, hindering the growth process.

However, it is important to note that everyone's hair is unique, and some individuals may need to adjust their washing routine accordingly. For instance, if you have an oily scalp, you may need to wash your hair more frequently to prevent excess sebum buildup, which can clog hair follicles and impede growth. On the other hand, if you have dry or curly hair, washing less frequently can help retain moisture and prevent frizz.

In addition to the frequency of washing, the choice of cleaning methods and products can also impact hair growth. Opt for gentle shampoos and conditioners that are free from harsh chemicals, sulfates, and parabens. These chemicals can strip away natural oils and cause damage to your hair, hindering its growth potential. Instead, consider using natural remedies such as homemade hair masks, herbal rinses, and essential oils to nourish and stimulate your scalp.

Lastly, maintaining a balanced and nutritious diet plays a vital role in promoting fast hair growth. Incorporate foods rich in vitamins, proteins, and minerals, such as leafy greens, eggs, fish, nuts, and seeds, into your daily meals. These nutrients provide the building blocks for strong and healthy hair, encouraging faster growth.

By understanding the optimal frequency of washing your hair, using gentle cleaning methods, and nourishing your body from within, you can maximize your hair growth potential. Remember, patience and consistency are key when it comes to achieving fast hair growth. With the right techniques, natural remedies, and nutritional foods, you can embark on a journey towards luscious, vibrant, and fast-growing hair.

Tips for Proper Hair Washing Techniques

Proper hair washing techniques play a crucial role in promoting fast hair growth. Many people underestimate the importance of this routine and end up damaging their hair unknowingly. In this subchapter, we will explore some essential tips that will help you achieve strong and healthy hair by adopting the right hair washing techniques.

1. Choosing the Right Shampoo: The first step towards proper hair washing is selecting the right shampoo. Look for a shampoo that suits your hair type and addresses any specific concerns you may have, such as dryness, dandruff, or oily scalp. Avoid shampoos containing harsh chemicals that can strip your hair of its natural oils.

2. Pre-Washing Preparation: Before jumping into the shower, it's essential to brush your hair gently to remove any tangles or knots. This helps prevent breakage during washing. Additionally, consider doing a pre-wash treatment with natural oils like coconut or olive oil to nourish and protect your hair.

3. Water Temperature: Use lukewarm or cool water to wash your hair instead of hot water. Hot water can strip away natural oils and leave your scalp dry. Coldwater, on the other hand, helps seal the hair cuticles, making your hair appear smoother and shinier.

4. Scalp Massage: While washing your hair, take a few extra minutes to give yourself a relaxing scalp massage. This stimulates blood flow to the hair follicles, promoting faster hair growth. Using your fingertips, gently massage your scalp in circular motions to relieve tension and enhance nutrient absorption.

5. Proper Technique: When applying shampoo, focus on the scalp rather than the lengths of your hair. Gently massage the shampoo into your scalp using your fingertips, ensuring it reaches the roots. Avoid using excessive force or rubbing vigorously, as this can damage the hair shafts and lead to breakage.

6. Conditioning: After rinsing off the shampoo, apply a conditioner to the lengths and ends of your hair. This helps restore moisture and detangles your hair, making it more manageable. Leave the conditioner on for a few minutes before rinsing it off thoroughly.

7. Drying: Avoid rubbing your hair vigorously with a towel. Instead, gently pat your hair dry to prevent unnecessary friction and breakage. Additionally, it's best to let your hair air dry naturally whenever possible, as excessive heat from blow dryers can damage the hair.

By following these tips for proper hair washing techniques, you can create an ideal environment for fast hair growth. Remember to be consistent with your routine, as healthy hair takes time to grow. Combine these techniques with proper nutrition and home remedies, as discussed in the rest of this book, and you'll be well on your way to achieving the long, luscious hair you desire.

Chapter 7: Additional Tips and Techniques for Fast Hair Growth

Protective Hairstyles for Hair Growth

One of the key factors in achieving fast hair growth is ensuring that your hair is well-protected and cared for. Protective hairstyles are an excellent way to promote hair growth while minimizing damage caused by everyday styling, environmental factors, and other external stressors. In this subchapter, we will explore a range of protective hairstyles that can help you on your journey to growing long and healthy hair.

1. Braids: Braiding your hair is a classic protective hairstyle that keeps your hair safe from tangles, breakage, and split ends. Whether you opt for box braids, cornrows, or French braids, this style helps to retain moisture and reduces manipulation, allowing your hair to grow undisturbed.

2. Buns and Updos: Keeping your hair in a bun or an updo not only looks elegant but also protects your hair from daily wear and tear. By securing your hair away from your face and shoulders, you prevent it from rubbing against clothing and getting tangled, leading to breakage.

3. Twists: Twists are another fantastic protective hairstyle that can promote hair growth. Whether you choose two-strand twists, three-strand twists, or even mini twists, this low-manipulation style helps to retain moisture and protect your hair from damage caused by external elements.

4. Wigs and Extensions: Wearing wigs or using hair extensions can be an effective way to protect your natural hair while allowing it to grow. These styles provide a protective barrier against heat, styling tools, and harsh weather conditions. Ensure that you maintain a healthy scalp by regularly cleansing and moisturizing your hair underneath.

5. Head Wraps and Scarves: If you're looking for a versatile and stylish way to protect your hair, head wraps and scarves are an excellent option. Not only do they shield your hair from damaging UV rays and pollution, but they also help to retain moisture and prevent breakage.

Remember, while protective hairstyles can encourage hair growth, it's equally important to maintain a healthy hair care routine alongside them. This includes regular washing, conditioning, and moisturizing, as well as incorporating essential nutrients into your diet.

By adopting protective hairstyles and practicing proper hair care, you can provide the ideal environment for your hair to grow quickly and healthily. Experiment with different styles, find what works best for you, and watch as your hair flourishes into the long, luscious locks you've always desired.

In the upcoming chapters, we will delve deeper into natural remedies, cleaning methods, and nutritional foods to complement your protective hairstyles and further accelerate your hair growth journey.

Avoiding Heat and Chemical Damage

One of the key factors that hinder fast hair growth is the damage caused by excessive heat and chemical treatments. In this subchapter, we will delve into the various ways you can avoid heat and chemical damage to promote healthy hair growth. By following these tips, you will be able to achieve the luscious, long locks you've always desired.

First and foremost, it is crucial to limit your use of heat styling tools such as flat irons, curling irons, and blow dryers. Excessive heat can strip your hair of its natural oils, leaving it dry, brittle, and prone to breakage. Whenever possible, embrace your hair's natural texture and allow it to air dry. If you must use heat styling tools, remember to always apply a heat protectant spray or serum to shield your strands from damage.

Chemical treatments like hair dyes, perms, and relaxers can also wreak havoc on your hair's health. These treatments often contain harsh chemicals that can weaken the hair shaft and lead to breakage. If you're looking to grow your hair quickly, it's best to avoid these treatments altogether. However, if you can't resist coloring your hair, opt for gentle, ammonia-free dyes and consider semi-permanent options that cause less damage.

In addition to avoiding heat and chemical treatments, it's essential to establish a proper hair care routine. Use shampoos and conditioners that are free from sulfates and parabens, as these ingredients can strip your hair of its natural moisture. Instead, opt for gentle, nourishing products that promote hair growth and repair.

Regular deep conditioning treatments are also paramount in maintaining healthy hair. These treatments help to replenish moisture, strengthen the hair shaft, and prevent breakage. Look for deep conditioners that contain natural ingredients such as coconut oil, shea butter, and argan oil. These oils are known for their moisturizing and repairing properties.

Lastly, protect your hair from the damaging effects of the sun and harsh weather conditions. UV rays can cause hair to become dry and brittle, so consider wearing a hat or using a UV protectant spray when spending time outdoors. During the winter months, shield your hair from the cold and dry air by wearing a hat or using a silk scarf as a protective barrier.

By following these tips and avoiding heat and chemical damage, you will pave the way for fast hair growth. Remember, patience and consistency are key when it comes to achieving the long, healthy hair you desire.

How to Deal with Hair Loss and Thinning

Hair loss and thinning can be a distressing experience for anyone, but the good news is that there are ways to address this issue and promote fast hair growth. In this subchapter, we will explore effective techniques and natural remedies to help you deal with hair loss and achieve the luscious locks you desire.

1. Understanding the Causes: Before diving into the solutions, it's important to understand the common causes of hair loss and thinning. From hormonal imbalances to nutritional deficiencies and stress, identifying the root cause will allow you to tailor your approach accordingly.

2. Home Remedies: There are several home remedies that can aid in hair growth. For instance, massaging your scalp with essential oils like rosemary or peppermint oil can stimulate hair follicles and improve blood circulation. Additionally, applying aloe vera gel or onion juice to your scalp can nourish the hair follicles and promote healthy hair growth.

3. Cleaning Methods: Proper hair cleaning techniques play a crucial role in maintaining a healthy scalp and encouraging hair growth. Avoid using harsh shampoos that strip away natural oils and opt for sulfate-free and gentle cleansers. Additionally, make sure to massage your scalp while washing to stimulate blood circulation and remove any build-up of dirt or product residue.

4. Nutritional Foods: A well-balanced diet is essential for healthy hair growth. Include foods rich in vitamins A, C, and E, as well as biotin, zinc, and iron. Leafy greens, fatty fish, nuts, seeds, and eggs are all great options to incorporate into your diet. You may also consider adding supplements like Biotin or Omega-3 fatty acids to support hair growth.

5. Lifestyle Changes: Stress and poor lifestyle choices can contribute to hair loss. Incorporate stress-reducing activities such as yoga, meditation, or regular exercise into your routine. Avoid excessive heat styling, tight hairstyles, and chemical treatments that can damage your hair.

6. Seek Professional Help: If your hair loss persists or worsens despite your efforts, it may be beneficial to consult a dermatologist or a trichologist. They can assess your condition and provide personalized treatment options such as medication, laser therapy, or hair transplants.

Remember, hair growth is a gradual process, and consistency is key. By implementing these techniques and natural remedies, you can take control of your hair health and achieve the fast hair growth you desire.

Chapter 8: Maintaining and Managing Fast Hair Growth

Trimming and Maintaining Hair Length

One of the key factors in achieving fast hair growth is proper trimming and maintenance. While it may seem counterintuitive to cut your hair when you're trying to grow it out, regular trims are essential for maintaining healthy hair length. This subchapter will provide you with valuable tips and techniques on how to trim and maintain your hair length effectively.

First and foremost, it's important to understand that split ends can hinder hair growth. Split ends occur when the protective cuticle of the hair shaft starts to wear away, causing the hair to split into two or more strands. To prevent further damage, it's crucial to trim your hair regularly to remove split ends. Aim to get a trim every 6-8 weeks, as this will help maintain your hair's overall health and encourage faster growth.

When it comes to trimming your hair, it's recommended to visit a professional stylist who specializes in hair growth. They will be able to assess the condition of your hair and provide a customized trim that promotes growth. Communicate your goals to the stylist, emphasizing that you want to maintain the length while removing any damaged ends.

In addition to professional trims, you can also perform maintenance trims at home. Invest in a good pair of hair shears and learn how to trim your hair yourself. Remember to use sharp, quality shears and follow a simple technique: take small sections of hair and trim off only the damaged ends. This way, you'll keep your hair length intact while removing split ends and promoting growth.

Alongside trimming, it's crucial to adopt a proper hair care routine to maintain the length and promote fast growth. This includes using a wide-toothed comb or a brush with gentle bristles to prevent breakage. Avoid excessive heat styling and use heat protectant products when necessary. Opt for sulfate-free shampoos and conditioners that are gentle on the hair. Additionally, incorporate deep conditioning treatments and hair masks into your routine to nourish and moisturize your hair, promoting healthy growth.

Remember, healthy hair starts from within. Integrate a balanced diet rich in essential vitamins and minerals, such as biotin, vitamin E, and omega-3 fatty acids. These nutrients support hair growth and overall hair health. Additionally, stay hydrated by drinking plenty of water to keep your hair moisturized from the inside out.

By following these tips on trimming and maintaining hair length, you'll be well on your way to achieving fast hair growth. Consistent trims, a proper hair care routine, and a healthy lifestyle will contribute to the long, luscious locks you desire.

Dealing with Split Ends and Breakage

Split ends and breakage can be a major hindrance when it comes to achieving fast hair growth. Not only do they make your hair look frizzy and unkempt, but they also prevent your hair from growing long and healthy. If you're looking to grow your head hair fast using home remedies, cleaning methods, and nutritional foods, it's essential to address the issue of split ends and breakage. In this subchapter, we will explore effective techniques and natural remedies to deal with these common hair problems.

One of the primary causes of split ends and breakage is excessive heat styling and chemical treatments. To protect your hair from damage, it's crucial to minimize the use of heat styling tools such as straighteners, curling irons, and blow dryers. When using these tools, always apply a heat protectant spray or serum to create a barrier between your hair and the heat. Additionally, opt for gentle and natural hair care products without harsh chemicals that can weaken the hair shaft and lead to breakage.

Regular trimming is another key strategy to combat split ends. While it may seem counterintuitive to cut your hair when you're trying to grow it out, trimming the ends every 6-8 weeks helps to remove split ends and prevent them from traveling up the hair shaft. This promotes healthier hair growth in the long run.

Incorporating natural remedies into your hair care routine can also work wonders in preventing split ends and breakage. Deep conditioning treatments with ingredients like coconut oil, argan oil, and honey provide nourishment and moisture to your hair, reducing the risk of breakage. Apply these treatments once or twice a week, leaving them on for at least 30 minutes before rinsing them out.

Another effective remedy for split ends is the use of protein treatments. Protein helps to strengthen the hair shaft and repair any damage, preventing breakage. Look for protein-rich hair masks or DIY treatments containing ingredients like eggs, yogurt, or mayonnaise. Apply these treatments once a month to maintain optimal hair health.

Lastly, a healthy diet rich in essential vitamins and minerals plays a crucial role in preventing split ends and promoting fast hair growth. Include foods such as leafy greens, nuts, seeds, fish, and eggs in your diet to provide your hair with the necessary nutrients it needs to grow long and strong.

By following these techniques and incorporating natural remedies into your hair care routine, you can effectively deal with split ends and breakage while promoting fast hair growth. Remember, patience and consistency are key, and with the right approach, you'll soon achieve the luscious, long hair you desire.

Styling Tips to Showcase Your Fast-Growing Hair

Congratulations on embarking on your journey to grow your head hair fast! In this subchapter, we will focus on styling tips that will not only showcase your fast-growing hair but also boost your confidence and make you feel fantastic. Whether you're attending a social event, heading to the office, or simply going about your daily routine, these tips will help you rock your new, luscious locks with style.

1. Embrace Layered Haircuts: Opt for layered haircuts that add depth and volume to your fast-growing hair. Layers create movement and make your hair appear fuller, giving it a healthy and vibrant look. Consult with a professional hairstylist who can suggest the best layering technique based on your hair type and face shape.

The Ultimate Guide to Fast Hair Growth: Proven Techniques and Natural Remedies

2. Experiment with Hair Accessories: Hair accessories are a great way to add flair and personality to your fast-growing hair. Try using headbands, hair clips, or stylish barrettes to jazz up your hairstyle. These accessories can help keep your hair in place while adding a touch of elegance or playfulness to your overall look.

3. Emphasize Your Natural Texture: If you're growing your hair fast, it's essential to embrace your natural texture. Let your curls, waves, or straight hair shine by using products specifically designed to enhance your hair's natural beauty. Embracing your natural texture not only saves time but also promotes healthy hair growth.

4. Master the Art of Braiding: Braids are a versatile and timeless hairstyle that can showcase the length and health of your fast-growing hair. Experiment with different braid styles like fishtail braids, French braids, or Dutch braids. Not only do braids look beautiful, but they also protect your hair from heat damage and breakage.

5. Play with Updos: Updos are a fantastic way to showcase your fast-growing hair while keeping it out of your face. Try different updo styles like buns, ponytails, or top knots. These hairstyles are not only practical but can also be customized to suit any occasion, from casual to formal events.

Remember, as you embark on your fast hair growth journey, it's crucial to maintain a healthy hair care routine. Regularly trim your hair to prevent split ends, nourish your hair with nutrient-rich products, and protect it from heat and environmental damage. By following these styling tips and incorporating them into your daily routine, you'll be able to showcase your fast-growing hair with confidence and style.

Chapter 9: Troubleshooting Hair Growth Issues

Identifying and Addressing Scalp Conditions

Subchapter: Identifying and Addressing Scalp Conditions

Introduction:

Taking care of your scalp is essential for promoting fast hair growth. A healthy scalp provides the right environment for your hair follicles to flourish and produce strong, voluminous hair. However, various scalp conditions can hinder hair growth and lead to hair loss. In this subchapter, we will explore the most common scalp conditions and provide effective techniques and natural remedies to address them. By understanding and treating these conditions, you can pave the way for fast hair growth.

1. Dandruff:

Dandruff is a common scalp condition characterized by dry, flaky skin. It can be caused by an overgrowth of yeast, dryness, or sensitivity to certain hair products. To address dandruff, you can try natural remedies such as tea tree oil, aloe vera, or apple cider vinegar rinses. Additionally, using a gentle shampoo formulated for dandruff and maintaining a clean scalp through regular cleansing can help alleviate this condition.

2. Scalp Psoriasis:

Psoriasis is a chronic autoimmune condition that affects the skin, including the scalp. It leads to red, scaly patches that can be itchy and uncomfortable. To manage scalp psoriasis, you can use natural remedies like coconut oil, aloe vera gel, or fish oil supplements. It is crucial to avoid scratching the affected areas and to consult a dermatologist for advanced treatment options if necessary.

3. Seborrheic Dermatitis:

Seborrheic dermatitis is a common scalp condition that causes redness, itching, and flaking. It is often associated with excessive oil production and the presence of a yeast called Malassezia. To address this condition, you can try home remedies like applying a mixture of apple cider vinegar and water, using aloe vera gel, or using shampoos containing ketoconazole or zinc pyrithione.

4. Hair Follicle Infections:

Infections such as folliculitis can cause inflammation and damage to the hair follicles, leading to hair loss. To prevent and treat these infections, it is essential to maintain good scalp hygiene, avoid sharing hair tools, and refrain from using heavy hair products that can clog the follicles. Additionally, natural remedies like tea tree oil or warm compresses can help alleviate the symptoms and promote healing.

Conclusion:

Identifying and addressing scalp conditions is crucial for achieving fast hair growth. By properly understanding these conditions and utilizing effective natural remedies, cleaning methods, and nutritional foods, you can create an optimal environment for your hair to thrive. Remember to consult a healthcare professional if your scalp condition persists or worsens. With diligence and care, you can pave the way for healthy, luscious hair.

Overcoming Hair Growth Plateaus

One of the most frustrating experiences when trying to grow long, luscious locks is hitting a plateau in hair growth. It often feels like no matter what you do, your hair just won't grow beyond a certain length. But fear not, for there are several effective techniques and natural remedies to help you overcome these hair growth plateaus and achieve the fast hair growth you desire.

First and foremost, it is essential to maintain a healthy scalp. A clean and well-nourished scalp provides the optimal environment for hair growth. Regularly cleanse your scalp using gentle shampoos and avoid excessive use of styling products that can clog hair follicles. Additionally, consider incorporating natural remedies like apple cider vinegar rinses or aloe vera gel massages to promote scalp health and stimulate hair growth.

Nutrition plays a vital role in hair growth as well. Ensure you are consuming a balanced diet rich in essential vitamins and minerals. Incorporate foods like leafy greens, eggs, nuts, and fatty fish into your meals, as they are packed with nutrients that support hair growth. If needed, consider incorporating hair growth supplements like biotin or collagen into your daily routine to provide your body with the necessary building blocks for healthy hair.

Regular hair care practices are also crucial in overcoming hair growth plateaus. Avoid excessive heat styling, as it can damage the hair shaft and hinder growth. Opt for air-drying whenever possible and use heat protectants when heat styling is necessary. Additionally, be gentle when detangling your hair to prevent breakage, and opt for wide-toothed combs or your fingers instead of harsh brushes.

Incorporating natural remedies into your hair care routine can provide an extra boost for fast hair growth. Consider using essential oils like rosemary, lavender, or peppermint, which have been known to stimulate hair growth. Dilute these oils with a carrier oil like coconut or jojoba oil and massage them into your scalp regularly.

Remember, consistency is key when it comes to overcoming hair growth plateaus. Incorporate these techniques and natural remedies into your daily routine and be patient. Rome wasn't built in a day, and neither is a head full of long, healthy hair. With dedication and perseverance, you can overcome those plateaus and achieve the fast hair growth you've always dreamed of.

Seeking Professional Help for Hair Growth Concerns

While home remedies, cleaning methods, and nutritional foods can be effective in promoting hair growth, there are instances where seeking professional help becomes necessary. If you have been struggling with hair growth concerns and have not seen any improvement despite your efforts, it may be time to consult professionals who specialize in hair care and restoration. In this subchapter, we will explore the benefits of seeking professional help and the various experts you can turn to for guidance.

One of the key advantages of consulting a professional is their expertise in diagnosing the underlying causes of your hair growth concerns. Hair loss or slow hair growth can be attributed to a variety of factors, including hormonal imbalances, genetic predisposition, nutritional deficiencies, scalp conditions, or even stress. By visiting a professional, you can receive a thorough assessment to determine the root cause of your hair growth issues. This knowledge is crucial in developing a personalized plan for effective hair growth.

When seeking professional help, you have several options to consider. Trichologists are specialists who focus on the health of the hair and scalp. They can provide valuable insights into your specific hair concerns and recommend suitable treatments, including topical solutions, medicated shampoos, or dietary supplements to address any deficiencies. Dermatologists, on the other hand, are medical doctors who specialize in skin, hair, and nail conditions. They can diagnose and treat any underlying medical conditions that may be affecting your hair growth.

Hair stylists and salon professionals can also provide assistance in your hair growth journey. They can offer advice on proper hair care practices, such as choosing the right products, avoiding damaging hairstyles or treatments, and maintaining a healthy scalp environment. Additionally, they can recommend techniques like scalp massages or laser therapy, which can stimulate hair follicles and promote growth.

While seeking professional help is essential, it is important to remember that it should complement your home remedies and natural remedies, not replace them. A holistic approach to hair growth combines the expertise of professionals with the power of natural remedies and self-care practices. By integrating both approaches, you can optimize your chances of achieving fast and healthy hair growth.

In conclusion, if you have been struggling to grow your head hair despite your best efforts, seeking professional help can provide valuable insights and solutions. Trichologists, dermatologists, and hair stylists are experts who can diagnose the underlying causes of your hair growth concerns, recommend suitable treatments, and guide you towards healthy hair practices. Remember to combine their expertise with your home remedies and natural remedies for a holistic approach to fast hair growth.

Chapter 10: Embracing and Celebrating Your Fast-Growing Hair

Boosting Confidence and Self-Esteem through Hair Growth

The Ultimate Guide to Fast Hair Growth: Proven Techniques and Natural Remedies

Having a head full of healthy, luscious hair can do wonders for your confidence and self-esteem. Whether you're dealing with hair loss, thinning hair, or simply want to accelerate the growth of your locks, this subchapter will provide you with proven techniques and natural remedies to boost hair growth and regain your confidence.

Hair loss or slow hair growth can be a frustrating experience, but with the right methods and a little patience, you can achieve remarkable results. In this subchapter, we will explore effective home remedies, cleaning methods, and nutritional foods that can help you grow your head hair fast.

Home remedies have long been used to promote hair growth, and many of them have stood the test of time. From scalp massages with essential oils to homemade hair masks using natural ingredients, we will discuss various techniques you can easily incorporate into your hair care routine. These methods not only stimulate hair growth but also improve the overall health of your scalp and hair follicles.

In addition to home remedies, maintaining a clean and healthy scalp is crucial for fast hair growth. We will delve into the importance of regular cleansing and share tips on how to properly clean your hair to remove product buildup and unclog hair follicles. By adopting the right cleaning methods, you can create an optimal environment for hair growth.

Furthermore, the food you consume plays a significant role in the health of your hair. We will explore a range of nutritional foods that are rich in vitamins and minerals essential for hair growth. From leafy greens to protein-rich foods, incorporating these into your diet can provide your body with the necessary nutrients to support fast hair growth.

Growing your head hair fast not only improves your physical appearance but also has a profound impact on your confidence and self-esteem. By following the techniques and remedies outlined in this subchapter, you will not only witness noticeable hair growth but also experience a newfound sense of confidence and self-assurance.

In conclusion, this subchapter is dedicated to providing you with the ultimate guide to fast hair growth. Whether you're looking to combat hair loss, increase hair thickness, or simply accelerate hair growth, the techniques and remedies discussed here will help you achieve your goals. With a little dedication and the right approach, you can boost your confidence and self-esteem through hair growth.

Embracing Your Natural Hair Texture

In the quest for fast hair growth, many of us tend to overlook the importance of embracing our natural hair texture. We often become fixated on specific hairstyles or trends, resorting to damaging treatments and excessive heat styling. However, it's crucial to realize that our hair's natural texture is beautiful and unique. By embracing it, we can actually promote healthier and faster hair growth.

Firstly, it's important to understand that each hair type has its own specific needs. Whether you have straight, wavy, curly, or kinky hair, there are specific techniques and remedies that can help you grow your hair faster. By understanding and working with your natural texture, you can optimize your hair growth potential.

For those with straight hair, one of the best ways to embrace your natural texture is by avoiding excessive heat styling and chemical treatments. Straight hair tends to be more prone to damage, so it's essential to protect it. Instead of using hot tools, try air-drying your hair or using low-heat methods to style it. Additionally, incorporating nourishing hair masks and adopting a healthy diet rich in vitamins and minerals can promote faster hair growth.

If you have wavy or curly hair, it's important to embrace your natural texture by avoiding excessive brushing or combing when your hair is dry. This can lead to breakage and frizz. Instead, try gently detangling your hair when it's wet, using a wide-toothed comb or your fingers. Embracing your natural waves or curls can lead to healthier hair growth and enhance your overall hair texture.

For those with kinky or coily hair, it's crucial to understand the unique needs of your hair type. Embrace your natural texture by using moisturizing products and protective styles that promote hair growth. Avoid harsh chemicals and excessive manipulation, as they can cause damage and hinder hair growth. Instead, focus on gentle detangling, deep conditioning, and nourishing your scalp to optimize your natural hair growth potential.

Regardless of your hair type, it's important to remember that your hair texture is beautiful and unique. By embracing it, you'll not only promote faster hair growth but also enhance the overall health and appearance of your hair. Embracing your natural hair texture is an essential step towards achieving your goal of fast hair growth, and it's a journey worth taking.

Sharing Your Hair Growth Journey with Others

One of the most rewarding aspects of embarking on a hair growth journey is the opportunity to share your progress and inspire others along the way. Whether you are using home remedies, exploring different cleaning methods, or incorporating nutritional foods into your diet, your journey can serve as a source of motivation and guidance for those looking to grow their head hair fast.

First and foremost, opening up about your hair growth journey creates a sense of camaraderie and support within the community. By sharing your experiences, struggles, and successes, you let others know that they are not alone in their quest for luscious locks. Through online platforms, social media groups, or even in-person discussions, you can connect with like-minded individuals who are also passionate about fast hair growth.

Furthermore, documenting your progress can be a powerful tool for both yourself and others. Consider starting a blog or vlog dedicated to your hair growth journey. This allows you to share your personal insights, techniques, and natural remedies with a wider audience. As you continue to update your platform regularly, you will not only keep yourself accountable but also provide valuable information and inspiration to others who are seeking effective hair growth methods.

Remember, your journey is unique and can serve as a valuable learning experience for others. Be sure to include any challenges you have faced and how you overcame them. This will help others avoid common pitfalls and provide them with the confidence to persevere through their own hair growth journey.

In addition to sharing your own experiences, it is important to actively engage with others who are on a similar path. Offer support, answer questions, and provide guidance whenever possible. By being an active participant in the hair growth community, you not only contribute to its growth but also benefit from the wealth of knowledge and shared experiences.

Finally, don't be afraid to display your before and after photos. Visual representations of your progress can be incredibly inspiring and encourage others to take action. Your transformation can serve as a testament to the effectiveness of the techniques and remedies you have employed, giving hope to those who may be skeptical or discouraged.

In conclusion, sharing your hair growth journey with others is a way to connect, inspire, and empower individuals who are eager to grow their head hair fast. By documenting your progress, providing insights, and actively engaging with the community, you contribute to a supportive network that helps others achieve their hair growth goals. Together, we can all achieve the fast hair growth we desire, using natural remedies, cleaning methods, and nutritional foods.

Conclusion: Achieving Fast Hair Growth and Maintaining Healthy Hair

In this guide, we have explored various proven techniques and natural remedies to help you achieve fast hair growth and maintain healthy hair. Whether you are looking to grow out your hair or simply improve its health, the information provided here will serve as a comprehensive resource for achieving your hair goals.

The Ultimate Guide to Fast Hair Growth: Proven Techniques and Natural Remedies

Firstly, we discussed the importance of understanding your hair type and identifying any underlying issues that may be hindering its growth. By recognizing factors such as dryness, brittleness, or dandruff, you can tailor your hair care routine to address these specific concerns.

We then delved into the world of home remedies, providing you with a range of effective solutions that can be easily prepared with ingredients found in your kitchen. From hair masks to scalp massages, these remedies have been proven to stimulate hair growth and nourish your locks from the roots.

Furthermore, we explored different cleaning methods that can contribute to fast hair growth. By adopting techniques such as co-washing, oil cleansing, or using natural shampoos and conditioners, you can minimize damage caused by harsh chemicals and promote a healthier scalp environment.

Nutrition plays a crucial role in hair growth, and we dedicated a section to highlight the importance of incorporating certain foods into your diet. From protein-rich sources to vitamins and minerals, these nutrients are essential for the production of healthy hair follicles and overall hair health.

To ensure long-term success in your hair growth journey, we emphasized the significance of maintaining a consistent hair care routine. Regular trimming, protecting your hair from heat and environmental damage, and avoiding tight hairstyles are all crucial steps to prevent hair breakage and promote healthy growth.

In conclusion, achieving fast hair growth and maintaining healthy hair requires a multi-faceted approach. By understanding your hair type, utilizing home remedies, adopting proper cleaning methods, and nourishing your body with the right nutrients, you can achieve the long and healthy hair you desire. Remember, consistency and patience are key, as hair growth is a gradual process that requires dedication and care. With the knowledge gained from this guide, you are now equipped to embark on your journey towards fast hair growth and vibrant, healthy locks.

www.ingramcontent.com/pod-product-compliance
Lightning Source LLC
Chambersburg PA
CBHW081500250726
48662CB00009B/3156